" The Growers
Journal to the
Coalesce."

- @wcfinest

Cannabis Grow Checklist

Plant Name   **Date Planted**

Water
Requirements 💧   💧💧   💧💧💧   Sunlight ☀ ☀ ●

☐ Seed   ☐ Transplant

Date	Event

Notes

Outcome

Uses

Purchased at: _________________________________   Price: _______________

January 2020

Sun	Mon	Tue	Wed	Thu	Fri	Sat
29	30	31	1	2	3	4
5	6	7	8	9	10	11
12	13	14	15	16	17	18
19	20	21	22	23	24	25
26	27	28	29	30	31	1

Cannabis Grow Checklist

Plant Name   **Date Planted**

Water
Requirements 🌢 🌢🌢 🌢🌢🌢   Sunlight ☀ ☀ ⚫

☐ Seed   ☐ Transplant

Date	Event

Notes

Outcome

Uses

Purchased at: ________________________   Price: ____________

February 2020

Sun	Mon	Tue	Wed	Thu	Fri	Sat
26	27	28	29	30	31	1
2	3	4	5	6	7	8
9	10	11	12	13	14	15
16	17	18	19	20	21	22
23	24	25	26	27	28	29

Cannabis Grow Checklist

Plant Name	**Date Planted**

Water
Requirements 💧 💧💧 💧💧💧　　　　Sunlight ☀ ☀ ●

☐ Seed　　　☐ Transplant

Date	Event

Notes

Outcome

Uses

Purchased at: ________________________　　Price: ________________

March 2020

Sun	Mon	Tue	Wed	Thu	Fri	Sat
1	2	3	4	5	6	7
8	9	10	11	12	13	14
15	16	17	18	19	20	21
22	23	24	25	26	27	28
29	30	31	1	2	3	4

Cannabis Grow Checklist

Plant Name	**Date Planted**

Water
Requirements 💧 💧💧 💧💧💧   Sunlight ☼ ☼ ●

☐ Seed   ☐ Transplant

Date	Event

Notes

Outcome

Uses

Purchased at: _______________________   Price: _______________________

April 2020

Sun	Mon	Tue	Wed	Thu	Fri	Sat
29	30	31	1	2	3	4
5	6	7	8	9	10	11
12	13	14	15	16	17	18
19	20	21	22	23	24	25
26	27	28	29	30	1	2

Cannabis Grow Checklist

Plant Name   **Date Planted**

Water
Requirements 💧 💧💧 💧💧💧   Sunlight ☀ ◐ ●

☐ Seed   ☐ Transplant

Date	Event

Notes

Outcome

Uses

Purchased at: _______________________________   Price: _______________

May 2020

Sun	Mon	Tue	Wed	Thu	Fri	Sat
26	27	28	29	30	1	2
3	4	5	6	7	8	9
10	11	12	13	14	15	16
17	18	19	20	21	22	23
24	25	26	27	28	29	30
31	1	2	3	4	5	6

Cannabis Grow Checklist

Plant Name	**Date Planted**

Water Requirements 💧 💧💧 💧💧💧

Sunlight ☼ ◑ ●

☐ Seed ☐ Transplant

Date	Event

Notes

Outcome

Uses

Purchased at: _______________________ Price: _______________________

June 2020

Sun	Mon	Tue	Wed	Thu	Fri	Sat
31	1	2	3	4	5	6
7	8	9	10	11	12	13
14	15	16	17	18	19	20
21	22	23	24	25	26	27
28	29	30	1	2	3	4

Cannabis Grow Checklist

Plant Name	**Date Planted**

Water Requirements 💧 💧💧 💧💧💧   Sunlight ☀ ☀ ●

☐ Seed   ☐ Transplant

Date	Event

Notes

Outcome

Uses

Purchased at: ___________________________   Price: ___________________

July 2020

Sun	Mon	Tue	Wed	Thu	Fri	Sat
28	29	30	1	2	3	4
5	6	7	8	9	10	11
12	13	14	15	16	17	18
19	20	21	22	23	24	25
26	27	28	29	30	31	1

Cannabis Grow Checklist

Plant Name   **Date Planted**

Water
Requirements   💧   💧💧   💧💧💧   Sunlight ☀ ☀ ⬤

☐ Seed   ☐ Transplant

Date	Event

Notes

Outcome

Uses

Purchased at: ______________________________   Price: ______________

August 2020

Sun	Mon	Tue	Wed	Thu	Fri	Sat
26	27	28	29	30	31	1
2	3	4	5	6	7	8
9	10	11	12	13	14	15
16	17	18	19	20	21	22
23	24	25	26	27	28	29
30	31	1	2	3	4	5

Cannabis Grow Checklist

Plant Name   **Date Planted**

Water
Requirements 🌢 🌢🌢 🌢🌢🌢   Sunlight ☀ ◐ ●

☐ Seed   ☐ Transplant

Date	Event

Notes

Outcome

Uses

Purchased at: _________________________   Price: _______________

September 2020

Sun	Mon	Tue	Wed	Thu	Fri	Sat
30	31	1	2	3	4	5
6	7	8	9	10	11	12
13	14	15	16	17	18	19
20	21	22	23	24	25	26
27	28	29	30	1	2	3

Cannabis Grow Checklist

Plant Name   **Date Planted**

Water
Requirements   🌢   🌢🌢   🌢🌢🌢   Sunlight   ☼ ☼ ⬤

☐ Seed   ☐ Transplant

Date	Event

Notes

Outcome

Uses

Purchased at: ______________________________   Price: ______________

October 2020

Sun	Mon	Tue	Wed	Thu	Fri	Sat
27	28	29	30	1	2	3
4	5	6	7	8	9	10
11	12	13	14	15	16	17
18	19	20	21	22	23	24
25	26	27	28	29	30	31

Cannabis Grow Checklist

Plant Name   **Date Planted**

Water
Requirements 💧 💧💧 💧💧💧   Sunlight

☐ Seed   ☐ Transplant

Date	Event

Notes

Outcome

Uses

Purchased at: ______________________________   Price: ______________

November 2020

Sun	Mon	Tue	Wed	Thu	Fri	Sat
1	2	3	4	5	6	7
8	9	10	11	12	13	14
15	16	17	18	19	20	21
22	23	24	25	26	27	28
29	30	1	2	3	4	5

Cannabis Grow
Checklist

Plant Name   **Date Planted**

Water
Requirements 🌢 🌢🌢 🌢🌢🌢   Sunlight ☀ ☀ ⚫

☐ Seed   ☐ Transplant

Date	Event

Notes

Outcome

Uses

Purchased at: _______________________   Price: _______________

December 2020

Sun	Mon	Tue	Wed	Thu	Fri	Sat
29	30	1	2	3	4	5
6	7	8	9	10	11	12
13	14	15	16	17	18	19
20	21	22	23	24	25	26
27	28	29	30	31	1	2

Strain

Grower

Date

Acquired

$

| Indica | Hybrid | Sativa |

☐ Flower   ☐ Edible   ☐ Concentrate

Symptoms Relieved

Notes

Sweet

Fruity

Floral

Sour

Spicy

Earthy

Herbal

Woodsy

Effects	Strength
Peaceful	○ ○ ○ ○ ○
Sleepy	○ ○ ○ ○ ○
Pain Relief	○ ○ ○ ○ ○
Hungry	○ ○ ○ ○ ○
Uplifted	○ ○ ○ ○ ○
Creative	○ ○ ○ ○ ○

Ratings ☆ ☆ ☆ ☆ ☆

2020

January

S	M	T	W	T	F	S
			1	2	3	4
5	6	7	8	9	10	11
12	13	14	15	16	17	18
19	20	21	22	23	24	25
26	27	28	29	30	31	

February

S	M	T	W	T	F	S
						1
2	3	4	5	6	7	8
9	10	11	12	13	14	15
16	17	18	19	20	21	22
23	24	25	26	27	28	29

March

S	M	T	W	T	F	S
1	2	3	4	5	6	7
8	9	10	11	12	13	14
15	16	17	18	19	20	21
22	23	24	25	26	27	28
29	30	31				

April

S	M	T	W	T	F	S
			1	2	3	4
5	6	7	8	9	10	11
12	13	14	15	16	17	18
19	20	21	22	23	24	25
26	27	28	29	30		

May

S	M	T	W	T	F	S
					1	2
3	4	5	6	7	8	9
10	11	12	13	14	15	16
17	18	19	20	21	22	23
24	25	26	27	28	29	30
31						

June

S	M	T	W	T	F	S
	1	2	3	4	5	6
7	8	9	10	11	12	13
14	15	16	17	18	19	20
21	22	23	24	25	26	27
28	29	30				

July

S	M	T	W	T	F	S
			1	2	3	4
5	6	7	8	9	10	11
12	13	14	15	16	17	18
19	20	21	22	23	24	25
26	27	28	29	30	31	

August

S	M	T	W	T	F	S
						1
2	3	4	5	6	7	8
9	10	11	12	13	14	15
16	17	18	19	20	21	22
23	24	25	26	27	28	29
30	31					

September

S	M	T	W	T	F	S
		1	2	3	4	5
6	7	8	9	10	11	12
13	14	15	16	17	18	19
20	21	22	23	24	25	26
27	28	29	30			

October

S	M	T	W	T	F	S
				1	2	3
4	5	6	7	8	9	10
11	12	13	14	15	16	17
18	19	20	21	22	23	24
25	26	27	28	29	30	31

November

S	M	T	W	T	F	S
1	2	3	4	5	6	7
8	9	10	11	12	13	14
15	16	17	18	19	20	21
22	23	24	25	26	27	28
29	30					

December

S	M	T	W	T	F	S
		1	2	3	4	5
6	7	8	9	10	11	12
13	14	15	16	17	18	19
20	21	22	23	24	25	26
27	28	29	30	31		

Made in the USA
Monee, IL
07 July 2026

56550093R00069